# Chair Yoga for Seniors Over 60 to Lose Weight

## 28-Day Weight Loss Challenge + BONUS: Audiobook and Video Courses

Carol Bolden

Copyright © 2024 by Carol Bolden



*Printed in USA*

*First Edition: Feb, 2024*

# Here is one of the biggest bonuses I promised you…

A full Audiobook on the **Chair Yoga for Seniors Over 60 to Lose Weight**

**To get access to it, kindly type in this link on your browser:**

http://tinyurl.com/5yks3khj

OR

**Scan the below QR code to gain access.**

**GET THE COMPLETE VIDEO COURSES AT THE END OF THIS BOOK**

# Table Of Content

# Introduction

In a world where the hustle and bustle of daily life can make it hard to find time for self-care, we often forget the importance of staying active and healthy. For seniors over 60, the challenge is even more significant, as the risk of injury and the need for specialized exercises can make regular fitness routines seem daunting. But fear not, for we have the perfect solution: Chair Yoga for Seniors Over 60 to Lose Weight.

This revolutionary 28-day weight loss challenge combines the ancient practice of yoga with modern-day scientific knowledge to create a safe, effective, and enjoyable way to shed those extra pounds, increase flexibility, and improve overall health. The best part? You can do it all from the comfort of a chair! No more worrying about balance or straining your joints, as this program is specifically designed for seniors who want to stay active and healthy without risking injury.

In this comprehensive guide, you'll find everything you need to embark on this life-changing journey. From detailed instructions and step-by-step photos to expert advice and motivational tips, we've got you covered. Our 28-day challenge is tailored to your needs and abilities, ensuring that you'll see real results without feeling overwhelmed or discouraged.

But don't just take our word for it. Countless seniors have already experienced the incredible benefits of chair yoga, including weight loss, increased flexibility, and improved overall health. Take, for example, 65-year-old Linda from Florida, who lost 15 pounds and regained her energy and confidence after completing our 28-day challenge. Or 71-year-old John from California, who was able to reduce his joint pain and improve his balance, making everyday tasks much easier.

So, what are you waiting for? Join the thousands of seniors who have already transformed their lives with Chair Yoga for Seniors Over 60 to Lose Weight: The Ultimate 28-Day Weight Loss Challenge. Say goodbye to the stress and frustration of traditional weight loss programs, and say hello to a healthier, happier, and more vibrant you. Are you prepared to make the first move? The path to a new you begins right now!

## What is Chair Yoga?

So, you're curious about Chair Yoga, eh? Well, let me tell you, it's not just for the birds! Chair Yoga is a form of yoga that's been adapted to be more accessible for those who might have trouble with traditional yoga poses. It's like yoga for the rest of us, no pretzel-twisting required!

In Chair Yoga, you perform modified yoga poses while seated in a chair or using the chair for support. This makes it a great option for seniors, people with disabilities or injuries, or anyone who spends a lot of time sitting at a desk. It's like a yoga party, and everyone's invited!

Plus, it's a great way to sneak some exercise into your day without even having to leave your chair. So, next time you're feeling stiff from sitting at your computer all day, why not give Chair Yoga a try? Your body (and your boss) will thank you!

## Benefits of Chair Yoga for Seniors

***Improved Flexibility:*** Chair yoga helps seniors to stretch their muscles and increase flexibility, making it easier to perform daily tasks and reducing the risk of injury.

***Enhanced Strength:*** Chair yoga involves gentle movements that help seniors to build strength in their muscles, which is important for maintaining balance and preventing falls.

***Better Balance and Posture:*** Chair yoga helps seniors to improve their balance and posture by strengthening the muscles that support the spine and promoting proper alignment of the body.

***Reduced Stress and Anxiety:*** Chair yoga incorporates breathing exercises and meditation, which can help to reduce stress and anxiety, promoting a sense of calm and well-being.

***Increased Circulation:*** Chair yoga can help to improve blood flow and circulation, which is important for maintaining heart health and preventing blood clots.

***Pain Management:*** Chair yoga can help to alleviate pain and discomfort associated with conditions such as arthritis and fibromyalgia by promoting relaxation and reducing muscle tension.

***Social Interaction:*** Many seniors enjoy participating in chair yoga classes, which provide an opportunity to socialize and connect with others, promoting a sense of community and belonging.

Overall, chair yoga is a gentle and accessible form of exercise that offers numerous benefits for seniors, helping them to stay active, healthy, and engaged in their daily lives.

## Importance of Exercise for Seniors Over 60

Exercise is crucial for seniors over 60 as it can help improve overall health, reduce the risk of chronic diseases, and enhance the quality of life. Regular physical activity can help maintain muscle strength and flexibility, improve balance and coordination, and promote better cardiovascular health.

*Some of the specific benefits of exercise for seniors over 60 include:*

***Improved cardiovascular health:*** Regular exercise can help improve heart health by reducing blood pressure, increasing circulation, and lowering the risk of heart disease and stroke.

***Enhanced mobility and balance:*** Exercise can help improve muscle strength and flexibility, which can improve mobility and balance, reducing the risk of falls and injuries.

***Better mental health:*** Exercise has been shown to have a positive impact on mental health, reducing the risk of depression and anxiety, and improving cognitive function and overall well-being.

***Increased bone density:*** Weight-bearing exercise can help improve bone density, reducing the risk of osteoporosis and fractures.

***Reduced risk of chronic diseases:*** Regular exercise can help reduce the risk of chronic diseases such as diabetes, obesity, and certain types of cancer.

# Chapter 1: Getting Started with Chair Yoga

## Choosing the Right Chair

Now, before we dive into the nitty-gritty of chair selection, let's take a moment to appreciate the fact that you've decided to engage in chair yoga. It's like a cosmic dance between you and the chair, a beautiful union of you and furniture.

But not all chairs are created equal, and the right chair can make all the difference in your practice. Here are the key factors to consider when choosing the best chair for your chair yoga sessions:

## Stability:

First and foremost, your chair must be stable. Imagine trying to find your center while sitting on a wobbly chair – it's like trying to find a needle in a haystack, only the needle is your inner peace, and the haystack is a world of distractions. So, make sure the chair has sturdy legs and a strong frame.

## Height:

Next, consider the height of the chair. Ideally, your feet should rest flat on the floor, with your knees bent at a 90-degree angle. This will help you maintain proper alignment and prevent any unnecessary strain on your back and legs. If your chair is too high, you might feel like you're trying to reach for the stars while practicing your chair yoga – and while that may be a noble pursuit, it's not exactly conducive to a grounded practice.

## Comfort:

Comfort is crucial, as you'll be spending a considerable amount of time in your chair. Look for a chair with a comfortable seat and backrest. A well-cushioned seat will provide support and prevent any discomfort during your practice. And a chair with a contoured backrest will offer additional support to your spine, making it easier to maintain proper posture.

## Armrests:

Armrests can be a double-edged sword. On one hand, they can provide additional support and help you maintain balance during certain poses. On the other hand, they can limit your range of motion and prevent you from fully exploring certain movements. If you decide to go for a chair with armrests, make sure they are removable or can be easily flipped up.

## Material:

The material of your chair is another important consideration. Look for a chair with a breathable fabric that allows air to circulate, keeping you cool and comfortable during your practice. A chair with a non-slip surface is also a good idea, as it will help you maintain your grip and prevent any unwanted sliding.

## Portability:

If you're a yoga nomad, always on the move, you'll want a chair that's easy to transport. Look for a lightweight chair that can be folded or disassembled for easy storage and transport. This way, you can take your chair yoga practice with you wherever you go, spreading joy and enlightenment to all corners of the galaxy.

## Style:

Finally, let's not forget about the importance of style. After all, your chair is an extension of your personality, and you want to make sure it reflects your unique sense of fashion. Choose a chair that speaks to you, one that makes you feel like a cosmic warrior embarking on a quest for inner peace and enlightenment.

# Creating a Safe Environment

Creating a safe environment for chair yoga exercises is essential for a comfortable and enjoyable practice. Here are some tips to help you create a safe space for your chair yoga sessions:

***Choose the right chair:*** Opt for a sturdy, stable chair with a straight back and no wheels. A chair with armrests can provide additional support during certain poses. Make sure the chair is the right height for you, allowing your feet to be flat on the floor and your knees bent at a 90-degree angle.

***Clear the space:*** Ensure that the area around your chair is free from clutter and obstacles. This will help prevent accidents and allow you to move freely during your practice.

***Proper lighting:*** Make sure your practice area is well-lit, so you can see clearly and maintain proper alignment during your poses.

***Proper ventilation:*** Good air circulation is important for maintaining a comfortable environment during your practice. Open a window or use a fan to ensure the room is well-ventilated.

***Temperature control:*** Keep the room at a comfortable temperature to prevent overheating or feeling cold during your practice.

***Minimize distractions:*** Create a calm and quiet atmosphere by turning off electronic devices, closing the door, and minimizing external noise. This will assist you in practicing with awareness and concentration.

***Use props:*** If you need additional support during your practice, consider using props such as cushions, blankets, or yoga blocks. These can help improve your alignment and make your practice more comfortable.

***Listen to your body:*** Always listen to your body and respect your limits. If something feels uncomfortable or painful, stop and adjust or skip the pose.

***Consult a professional:*** If you have any pre-existing conditions or concerns, consult with a healthcare professional or a qualified yoga instructor before starting your practice.

## Setting Realistic Goals

## Step 1: Assess your current fitness level

Before setting your goals, it's important to understand your starting point. Take a moment to assess your current fitness level. Are you a beginner with no prior yoga experience? Or do you have some experience with yoga but are new to chair yoga? You can establish more reasonable objectives if you are aware of where you stand.

## Step 2: Choose your goals

Now that you have a better understanding of your current fitness level, it's time to choose your goals. Start with small, achievable goals that will help you build confidence and motivation. For example, if you're a beginner, your goal might be to practice chair yoga for 15 minutes a day, three times a week. As you progress, you can increase the length and frequency of your practice.

## Step 3: Divide your objectives into manageable chunks.

Breaking your goals into smaller steps can make them feel more manageable and achievable. For example, if your goal is to practice chair yoga for 15 minutes a day, three times a week, you could break this down into daily goals. Start with five minutes of practice a day, and gradually increase the time as you become more comfortable with the exercises.

## Step 4: Create a plan

Now that you have your goals and smaller steps, it's time to create a plan. Set a schedule for your chair yoga practice, and stick to it as best you can. If you find that you're struggling to stick to your plan, don't be afraid to adjust it. Recall that progress, not perfection, is the aim.

## Step 5: Track your progress

As you work towards your goals, it's important to track your progress. Keep a journal or log of your practice, noting the exercises you do, the time you spend practicing, and how you feel. This will help you see how far you've come and give you a sense of accomplishment as you reach your goals.

# Chapter 2: Week 1: Gentle Movements for Mobility

## Day 1

## Seated Cat-Cow Stretch

- Place your hands on your thighs and your feet flat on the floor as you sit in a chair. Ensure that your shoulders are relaxed and your back is straight.
- Take a deep breath and arch your back, pushing your chest forward and your shoulder blades back. This is the "cow" position.
- As you exhale, round your back and tuck your chin towards your chest, creating a "cat" position.
- Continue alternating between these two positions, moving with your breath. Inhale for cow and exhale for cat.
- Repeat this sequence for 10-15 breaths, or as long as it feels comfortable and beneficial for you.

## Seated Forward Bend

The Seated Forward Bend, also known as Paschimottanasana, is a fantastic yoga pose to stretch your hamstrings and lower back while calming your mind. Here's a step-by-step guide to help you master this pose:

***Preparation:***

- To practice, choose a place that is peaceful and cozy.
- Put on loose, comfortable apparel that doesn't restrict your range of motion.
- Choose a yoga mat or a soft surface to sit on.

***Starting Position:***

- With your legs out in front of you, take a seat on the floor.

- Place your hands on the floor beside your hips, palms facing down.
- Align your spine, shoulders relaxed, and chest lifted.

### *Bending Forward:*

- Inhale deeply, and as you exhale, gently bend forward from your hips.
- Maintain a long spine and relaxed shoulders.
- Reach your hands towards your feet or ankles, or hold onto your calves or thighs if you can't reach your feet.
- If you can't reach your feet, use a yoga strap or a towel to loop around your feet and hold onto the ends.

### *Hold the Pose:*

- Hold the Seated Forward Bend for 1 to 3 minutes, breathing deeply and evenly.
- Focus on relaxing your body and deepening the stretch with each exhale.
- If you feel any discomfort or pain, gently release the pose and rest in a comfortable position.

### *Release and Relax:*

- To release the pose, slowly inhale and come back to a seated position, keeping your spine long.
- Exhale and relax your shoulders.
- Take a moment to feel the effects of the pose and enjoy the relaxation.

## Seated Spinal Twist

- With your legs out in front of you, take a seat on the floor. If you have tight hamstrings or lower back pain, you can sit on a folded blanket or a yoga block to elevate your hips.
- Bend your right knee and place your right foot on the outside of your left knee.

- For support, place your left hand on the ground behind you.
- Inhale and lift your right arm up towards the sky, extending your spine and opening your chest.
- Exhale and twist your torso to the right, placing your right hand on the outside of your left knee or on the floor beside your left hip.
- Maintain a long spine and relaxed shoulders.
- Press your right fingertips into the floor or your left knee to deepen the twist.
- After five to ten breaths, hold the stance, then release it and switch to the opposite side.

## Seated Side Stretch

- Sit on a chair with your feet flat on the ground and your back straight.
- Inhale deeply and raise your right arm up towards the sky, extending your spine and opening your chest.
- Exhale and lean your torso to the left, stretching from the hip bone to the tips of your fingers. Place your left hand on the chair for support or rest it on your left thigh.
- Hold the stretch for 3 breaths, feeling the stretch along the right side of your body.
- Inhale and return to the center, then exhale and repeat the stretch on the other side.
- Perform 3-5 stretches on each side, or as many as feels comfortable for you.

## Seated Mountain Pose

- Sit on a chair with your feet flat on the ground and your back straight.
- With your palms facing down, place your hands on your thighs or knees.
- Take a deep breath and lift your chest, rolling your shoulders back and down.
- Keep your head forward and your chin parallel to the floor.
- Hold the pose for a few breaths, feeling your spine lengthen and your chest open.
- Exhale and release, returning to a relaxed seated position.

Day 2

## Seated Chair Pose

Step 1: Sit on a chair with your feet flat on the floor, hip-width apart.

Step 2: Place your hands on your thighs, palms facing down.

Step 3: Inhale deeply and lift your arms up towards the ceiling, extending your spine and opening your chest.

Step 4: Exhale and bend your knees, lowering your hips as if you're sitting back into an imaginary chair. Keep your arms parallel to your ears.

Step 5: Feel the stretch in your ankles, hips, and thighs as you hold the posture for three to five breaths.

Step 6: Breathe in, raise your hips back to the beginning position, and gradually straighten your legs. After exhaling, bring your arms down to your sides.

Step 7: Hold the position three to five times, or as often as it is comfortable for you.

## Seated Leg Lifts

- With your feet level on the ground and your back straight, take a seat on the edge of a solid chair.
- For support, rest your hands on the chair's sides.
- Maintaining your leg straight and stretched in front of you, raise one off the ground.
- After a brief period of holding the posture, return your leg to its initial position.

- With the second leg, do the exercise again.
- Once you reach the appropriate amount of repetitions, keep switching up the legs.

## Seated Arm Raises

- With your feet level on the ground and your back straight, take a seat on the edge of a solid chair.
- For support, rest your hands on the chair's sides.
- Stretch one arm straight out in front of you and raise it toward the sky.
- After a little while, hold the pose, then bring your arm back down to the beginning position.
- With the opposite arm, do the exercise again.
- For the necessary number of repetitions, keep switching arms.

## Seated Chair Dips

- Grasp the edges of a strong chair with your hands while sitting on its edge, pointing your fingers forward.
- Maintaining straight arms and flat feet on the floor, slide your butt off the chair's edge.
- Keep your back close to the chair as you lower your body by bending your elbows to a 90-degree angle.
- Contract your triceps and straighten your arms to push yourself back up to the starting position.
- For the required amount of repetitions, repeat.

## Seated Eagle Pose

- With your back straight and your feet flat on the floor, take a seat on a chair's edge.
- If it is feasible, place your right foot around your left calf and cross your right leg over your left leg.

- After crossing your left arm over your right arm at the elbow, encircle each other with your forearms, if at all possible bringing your palms together.
- As you sit up straight and take a big breath, notice how your shoulders and upper back are stretched.
- Take a few deep breaths to hold the stance, then release it and switch to the other side.

# Day 3

## Seated Chair Plank

- With your feet level on the floor and hip-width apart, take a seat on the edge of a solid chair.
- With your fingers pointed forward, grasp the seat with your hands on the chair's sides.
- Lean back a little while keeping your feet off the ground by using your core. Maintain erect limbs and pointed toes.
- Maintain this posture, being mindful to maintain a straight back and a contracted core.
- Try raising one leg at a time while keeping your balance for an extra challenge.
- You may hold the plank for a minute or thirty seconds, depending on your level of fitness.
- Release your hold on the chair and slowly drop your feet back to the ground.

## Seated Leg Extensions

- With your feet level on the ground and your back straight, take a seat on a chair.
- For support, rest your hands on the chair's sides.
- Maintaining your foot flexed and your leg straight, extend one leg out in front of you.
- After a brief period of holding the posture, return your leg to its initial position.
- With the second leg, do the exercise again.
- Once you reach the appropriate amount of repetitions, keep switching up the legs.

## Seated Leg Circles

- With your feet level on the ground and your back straight, take a seat on a chair's edge.
- Raise one leg straight up off the ground and place it in front of you.
- Keeping your toes pointing forward and your foot contracted, start creating little circles with your leg.
- Make ten to fifteen circles in one direction, then turn around and make another ten to fifteen circles in the other way.
- Return your leg to the floor, then use the other leg to complete the exercise.

## Seated Chair Crunches

- Place your feet level on the floor, hip-width apart, and take a seat on a chair's edge.
- With your elbows out to the sides, place your hands behind your head or on the chair's sides.
- Maintaining a straight back, contract your core and slant back slightly.
- Breathe out and use your abdominal muscles to contract as you raise your shoulders and upper back off the chair.
- Take a breath and come back to the beginning.
- After the specified amount of repetitions, repeat the crunch.

## Seated Tree Pose

- With your feet level on the floor and your back straight, take a seat on a chair to begin.
- Breathe deeply, then raise your right foot off the ground such that the inside of your left thigh is where the sole of your shoe is located.
- To establish a sensation of stability and anchoring, firmly press your left thigh into your right foot and your right foot into your left thigh.
- In a pose of prayer, place your hands near your heart. If you're feeling very daring, you may even extend your arms to the sky.
- Feel the stretch in your right hip and the activation of your core muscles as you hold the position for a few breaths.
- Repeat on the opposite side after letting go.

# Day 4

## Seated Butterfly Pose

- With your legs out in front of you, take a seat on the floor.
- Allowing your knees to drop to the sides, bend your knees, and bring the soles of your feet together.
- With your hands clasped around your feet or ankles, slowly bring your heels as near to your torso as feels comfortable.
- Maintain a straight spine and relaxed shoulders when sitting upright.
- After taking a deep breath, use your elbows to gently push your knees toward the floor.
- As you maintain the stance for 30 to 60 seconds, take slow, even breaths.
- Breathe gently in, elevate your knees, and then stretch your legs back in front of you to come out of the posture.

## Seated Head-to-Knee Pose

- The amazing yoga practice known as Janu Sirsasana, or Seated Head to Knee practice, serves to stretch the hamstrings, groins, and spine while also alleviating tension and soothing the mind. To assist you with this practice, follow these steps:
-
- Sit on the floor with your legs out in front of you to start; maintain a straight spine and relaxed shoulders.
- Gently push your right knee toward the floor while bending it and bringing the sole of your right foot up inside your left thigh.
- Taking a breath, raise your arms and extend them toward the sky. Breathe out, and then gradually start to bend forward from the hips, maintaining a long spine and a tight core.

- If you can, extend your hands to your left foot and grasp your left foot, ankle, or calf with them. If your foot is out of reach, you may close the distance with a towel or yoga strap.
- As you maintain the stance for 30 to 60 seconds, take slow, even breaths.
- Gently remove your hands off your left foot and return your body to an upright posture to exit the pose.
- On the opposite side, repeat the posture.

## Seated Half Lord of the Fishes Pose

Ardha Matsyendrasana, also known as the Seated Half Lord of the Fishes posture, is an amazing yoga posture that helps to relieve tension and stretch the hips, shoulders, and spine. To assist you with this practice, follow these steps:

- Sit on the floor with your legs out in front of you to start; maintain a straight spine and relaxed shoulders.
- With your right knee facing upwards, bend your right knee and place the sole of your right foot outside of your left knee.
- Breathe in, arching your back, opening your chest, and raising your left arm to the heavens.
- With your left elbow on the outside of your right knee and your right palm on the floor behind you for support, release your breath and rotate your body to the right.
- To increase the twist's depth, press your right fingers into the ground or your left knee.
- As you maintain the stance for 30 to 60 seconds, take slow, even breaths.
- Gently relax your torso and go back to the beginning posture to release the pose.
- On the opposite side, repeat the posture.

## Seated Wide-Legged Forward Bend

Upavistha Konasana, or the Seated Wide-Legged Forward Bend, is a fantastic yoga posture that helps to relieve tension and relax the mind in addition to stretching the spine, hamstrings, and groins. To assist you with this practice, follow these steps:

- Sit on the floor with your legs out in front of you to start; maintain a straight spine and relaxed shoulders.
- With your feet flexed and toes pointed upward, spread your legs as wide as feels comfortable for you.
- Taking a breath, raise your arms and extend them toward the sky. Breathe out and extend your hip flexion while maintaining a long spine and a tight core.
- If at all feasible, reach your hands down to your feet and use them to hold your ankles, calves, or feet. If you are unable to reach your feet, you may close the distance with a towel or yoga strap.
- As you maintain the stance for 30 to 60 seconds, take slow, even breaths.
- Gently remove your hands from your feet and return your body to an upright posture to exit the pose.

## Seated Bound Angle Pose

Baddha Konasana, or Seated Bound Angle practice, is a fantastic yoga practice that improves posture, stretches the lower back, and opens up the hips, groin, and inner thighs. To assist you with this practice, follow these steps:

- Sit on the floor with your legs out in front of you to start; maintain a straight spine and relaxed shoulders.
- Allowing your knees to drop to the sides, bend your knees, and bring the soles of your feet together.
- With your hands clasped around your feet or ankles, slowly bring your heels as near to your torso as feels comfortable.
- Maintain a straight spine and relaxed shoulders when sitting upright.
- After taking a deep breath, use your elbows to gently push your knees toward the floor.
- As you maintain the stance for 30 to 60 seconds, take slow, even breaths.

- Breathe gently in, elevate your knees, and then stretch your legs back in front of you to come out of the posture.

# Day 5

Repeat Day 1 Exercises

# Day 6

Repeat Day 2 Exercises

# Day 7

Repeat Day 3 Exercises

# Chapter 3: Week 2: Building Strength and Balance

Day 8

Repeat Day 4 Exercises

## Day 9

## Seated Chair Push-Ups

- With your feet level on the ground and shoulder-width apart, take a seat on the edge of a solid chair.
- Grasp the chair's edge with your hands, fingers pointing forward, just outside of your hips.
- Lean slightly forward while maintaining a straight back and relaxed shoulders by engaging your core.
- Bending your elbows and lowering your chest toward the chair can help you lower your body.
- Straighten your arms and push yourself back up to the starting position, maintaining a straight back and an engaged core.
- Continue till the desired number of times.

## Seated Chair Rows

- With your feet firmly planted on the floor and spaced shoulder-width apart, take a seat on a bench or chair.
- Bend over and place both hands, palms inside, on the cable row machine's grips.
- Maintain a straight back and a contracted core.
- After the action, squeeze your shoulder blades together while pulling the handles towards your body.

- Return the handles to their initial positions gradually while keeping your composure.
- Continue till the desired number of times.

## Seated Chair Reverse Fly

- With your feet flat on the floor and shoulder-width apart, take a seat on a bench or chair.
- Hold a dumbbell in each hand and stretch your arms at your sides, with the palms facing inward.
- Maintain a straight back and contract your core.
- Taking a deep breath, gradually extend your arms to the sides while maintaining a tiny bend in your elbows. At the peak of the action, squeeze your shoulder blades together.
- After holding the contraction for a few while, release the tension and gradually return the dumbbells to their initial position.
- Continue till the desired number of times.

## Seated Chair Curls

- With your feet flat on the floor and shoulder-width apart, take a seat on a chair.
- With your arms out at your sides and your palms facing outward, hold a dumbbell in each hand.
- Verify that your core is active and that your back is straight.
- Curl the dumbbells slowly in the direction of your shoulders, simply moving your forearms and not your upper arms.
- At the peak of the exercise, tighten your biceps, and then gradually drop the dumbbells back to the beginning position.
- Continue till the desired number of times.

## Seated Chair Tricep Extensions

- With your feet flat on the floor and shoulder-width apart, take a seat on a bench or chair.
- With your arms out at your sides and your palms facing inward, hold a dumbbell in each hand.
- Maintain a straight back and contract your core.
- Breathe in, then bend your elbows until the dumbbells are raised gently to a 90-degree angle.
- Take a breath out and raise your arms back up to the beginning position.
- Continue till the desired number of times.

# Day 10

## Seated Chair Squats

- With your feet level on the floor and shoulder-width apart, take a seat on a firm chair.
- Maintain a straight back and a contracted core.
- Breathe in and let your hips drop gradually as if you were reclining on a chair.
- After a brief period of holding the squat posture, release your breath and drive through your heels to go back to the beginning position.
- Continue till the desired number of times.

## Seated Chair Lunges

- With your feet level on the floor and shoulder-width apart, take a seat on a firm chair.
- Maintain a straight back and contract your core.
- Taking a deep breath, raise your right foot off the ground gradually while bringing your knee closer to your chest.
- With your foot flexed and toes pointed upward, release your breath and stretch your right leg in front of you.
- Breathe in, then gently return your right leg to the beginning position.
- After the required number of repetitions, swap legs and repeat.

## Seated Chair Calf Raises

- With your feet level on the floor and shoulder-width apart, take a seat on a firm chair.
- Lay a dumbbell or weight plate over your lap so that it rests between your thighs.
- To hold it stable, place your hands on the weight.

- Elevate your calves as high as possible while gradually lifting your heels off the ground.
- After a brief period of holding the contraction, gradually bring your heels back to the beginning position.
- Continue till the desired number of times.

## Seated Chair Hamstring Curls

- With your feet shoulder-width apart and your back straight, take a seat on a chair or bench.
- Keeping your arms straight, place a resistance band around the center of your feet and grasp both ends with both hands.
- Lift your heels slowly off the ground and bring your feet close to your glutes by tightening your hamstrings.
- After a few periods of holding the contraction, carefully return your heels to the beginning position.
- Continue till the desired number of times.

## Seated Chair Leg Swings

- With your feet level on the floor and shoulder-width apart, take a seat on a firm chair.
- For support, rest your hands on the chair's sides.
- Maintaining a straight back, contract your core and slant back slightly.
- With your foot flexed and toes pointed upward, raise one leg off the ground and swing it slowly forth and backward.
- After the required number of repetitions, swap legs and repeat.
- Try swinging both legs at the same time for extra difficulty.

## Day 11

Repeat Day 9 Exercises

Day 12

Repeat Day 10 Exercises

# Day 13

## Seated Chair Sun Salutations

Step 1: Find a solid chair that can hold your weight and serve as a solid base for your intergalactic journeys before setting off on your cosmic adventure.

Step 2: With your back to the seat, take a stance in front of the chair. Give yourself time to center and feel the energy of the cosmos flowing through you.

Step 3: Reach up toward the stars with your arms over your head and take a deep breath. Breathe out as you gently lean forward from your hips, maintaining a straight back, and rest your hands on the chair's seat.

Step 4: Breathe in, then raise your right leg back with the elegance of a thousand suns, bending your knee and planting the ball of your foot on the floor. Maintain both of your hands on the chair and your left foot firmly planted on the ground.

Step 5: Let out a breath and extend your left leg back to meet your right, bringing your torso parallel to the ground as you create a plank. Take a few deep breaths and maintain this posture, then channel the power of the universe.

Step 6: Breathe in and bring your knees, chest, and chin down to the floor with the force of a supernova. Breathe out and let your body fall to the ground as if you were giving yourself over to the boundless void.

Step 7: Take a breath, then raise your chest and straighten your arms by pressing your hands into the ground with the might of a thousand suns. Maintain your thighs and hips on the floor while looking ahead, as if you're trying to discover the universe's mysteries.

Step 8: Let out a breath and raise your hips and legs back into the plank posture with the elegance of a shooting star. Take a few deep breaths and hold this posture as you feel the energy of the universe pouring through you.

Step 9: Breathe in deeply, then raise your hips and bend your knees, bringing your feet back to the chair with the might of a thousand suns. Take a deep breath out, lift your hands off the chair, and stand back up.

Step 10: Breathe in, and raise your arms over your head, reaching for the stars, with the elegance of a thousand suns. After you release the air, bring your arms back to your sides and take a starting stance.

Step 11: Bask in the cosmic energy you have tapped into and experience your connection to the cosmos for a time. Follow the stars on your voyage by repeating this sequence as much as you want.

## Seated Chair Warrior Poses

Step 1: Locate a strong chair that can sustain your weight and your inner warrior's might.

Step 2: Assume a comfortable seated position on the chair's edge, keeping your feet firmly on the floor, and imagine that you are going to take off into space.

Step 3: Raise your chest and straighten your spine to embrace your inner warrior. Envision yourself as a powerful heavenly being, prepared to rule the cosmos.

Step 4: Take a deep breath and raise your arms to the sides, parallel to the floor, in the manner of someone preparing to embrace the immensity of the cosmos.

Step 5: Release the breath, bending your right arm and raising your palm to your chest in a toast to the stars. At the same time, stretch forward with your left arm, aiming for the stars. For a few breaths, hold this stance and feel the energy of the cosmos coursing through you.

Step 6: Take a breath, then go back to Step 4 and spread both arms out to the sides.

Step 7: Let out a breath and repeat Step 5 with your right arm extended and your left arm bent. For a few breaths, hold this stance and sense the inner harmony of the cosmos.

Step 8: Take a breath, then go back to Step 4 and spread both arms out to the sides.

Step 9: Let go and give yourself a cosmic hug by bringing both hands to your heart. Take a minute to experience the strength of your inner warrior and bathe in the energy of the cosmos.

Step 10: Continue doing this cosmic dance as often as you want, letting the universe's energy flow through you and direct you as you go.

## Seated Chair Triangle Pose

Step 1: Locate a strong chair that can sustain your weight and your inner warrior's might.

Step 2: Assume a comfortable seated position on the chair's edge, keeping your feet firmly on the floor, and imagine that you are going to take off into space.

Step 3: Raise your chest and straighten your spine to embrace your inner warrior. Envision yourself as a powerful heavenly being, prepared to rule the cosmos.

Step 4: Take a deep breath and raise your arms to the sides, parallel to the floor, in the manner of someone preparing to embrace the immensity of the cosmos.

Step 5: Release the breath, bending your right arm and raising your palm to your chest in a toast to the stars. At the same time, stretch forward with your left arm, aiming for the stars. For a few breaths, hold this stance and feel the energy of the cosmos coursing through you.

Step 6: Take a breath, then go back to Step 4 and spread both arms out to the sides.

Step 7: Let out a breath and repeat Step 5 with your right arm extended and your left arm bent. For a few breaths, hold this stance and sense the inner harmony of the cosmos.

Step 8: Take a breath, then go back to Step 4 and spread both arms out to the sides.

Step 9: Let go and give yourself a cosmic hug by bringing both hands to your heart. Take a minute to experience the strength of your inner warrior and bathe in the energy of the cosmos.

Step 10: Continue doing this cosmic dance as often as you want, letting the universe's energy flow through you and direct you as you go.

## Seated Chair Half Moon Pose

Step 1: Take a comfortable seat on the chair's edge and place your feet hip-width apart, flat on the ground.

Step 2: Tilt your upper body slightly to the right while placing your hands on your hips. Face forward with your legs and hips.

Step 3: Take a big breath in and extend your left arm straight up, aiming for the sky. Breathe out, tilt your head to the left, and gently stretch your left arm above your head.

Step 4: Feel the mild stretch in your left side as you hold the position for a few breaths.

Step 5: Take a breath, come back to the center, and lower your left arm to your side.

Step 6: Turn to the left and raise your right arm over your head while doing the identical movements on the other side.

Step 7: Switch sides for a few rounds while taking deep breaths and savoring the moon's energy.

## Seated Chair Pigeon Pose

Step 1: Place your feet firmly on the floor, hip-width apart, and sit up straight on the edge of a strong chair.

In the second step, inhale deeply and raise your right leg such that your right ankle rests on top of your left thigh. To protect your knee, make sure your right foot is flexed.

Step 3: Keeping your left foot firmly planted on the floor, use your right hand to gently push down on your right knee. Your right hip and glute will extend more deeply as a result.

Step 4: Feel the stretch in your right hip and glute as you hold this posture for five to ten deep breaths.

Step 5: You may gradually tilt forward from your hips to deepen the stretch while maintaining a long spine and raised chest. For a further five to ten breaths, hold this posture.

Step 6: Lower your right leg off your left thigh and plant your right foot back on the floor to release the stretch.

Step 7: Carry out the identical motions on the other side, pushing your left knee down with your left hand while raising your left ankle onto your right thigh.


## Day 14


Repeat Day 13 Exercises

# Please wait, Your Review is Very Important…

### *Dear Reader,*

I hope this message finds you well. Thank you for choosing to read the Chair Yoga for Seniors Over 60 to Lose Weight. Your feedback is incredibly valuable to me, and I would love to hear your thoughts on the book. Whether you've just started, are halfway through, or have finished reading, your perspective matters.

Your feedback is immensely appreciated and will help me enhance future works.

Thank you for taking the time to share your thoughts on Chair Yoga for Seniors Over 60 to Lose Weight. Your support means the world to me.

*Happy reading!*

Carol Bolden

# Chapter 4: Week 3: Deepening Your Practice

## Day 15

## Seated Chair Knee Tucks

Step 1: Take a comfortable seat on the chair's edge and place your feet hip-width apart, flat on the ground.

Step 2: Lift your chest and maintain a straight back while gently bending your back. This requires activating your core.

Step 3: Maintaining your left foot firmly on the ground, raise your right knee to your chest.

Step 4: Release your right leg back to the beginning position after holding the tuck for a little while.

Step 5: Tuck your left knee in again.

Step 6: Perform right and left knee tucks alternately for ten to fifteen repetitions on each side, or as many as you are comfortable with.

## Seated Chair Shoulder Press

Step 1: Place your feet level on the floor, hip-width apart, and settle into a comfortable seat on the edge of a strong chair with a backrest.

Step 2: With your elbows bent 90 degrees and your palms facing front, hold a dumbbell in each hand. Your forearms should be perpendicular to the floor, but your upper arms should be parallel to it.

Step 3: Maintain a straight back and contract your core.

Step 4: Let out a breath and raise the dumbbells with your arms extended completely. Avoid arching your back and maintain a neutral head and neck posture.

Step 5: Take a breath, hold the pose for a while, and then gradually bring the dumbbells back down to the beginning position.

Step 6: Complete the exercise as many times as you want. A single set usually consists of 8–12 repetitions.

## Seated Chair Chest Press

Step 1: Take a comfortable seat on the chair's edge and place your feet hip-width apart, flat on the ground.

Step 2: With your elbows bent 90 degrees and your palms facing front, hold a set of dumbbells at shoulder height.

Step 3: Breathe deeply and raise the dumbbells off your chest while putting your arms straight out in front of you. Breathe out while you do this.

Step 4: Inhale as you gently drop the dumbbells back to the beginning position after holding the posture for a little while.

Step 5: Perform the appropriate number of repetitions of the press and release exercise (for seniors, this is often 8–12 reps).

## Seated Chair Lat Pulldowns

Step 1: Take a comfortable seat on the chair's edge and place your feet hip-width apart, flat on the ground.

Step 2: Get a resistance band and wrap it around a bedpost or other solid item behind you. Ensure that it is firmly attached and raised to a level that permits a comfortable pulling action.

Step 3: With both hands, slightly wider than shoulder-width apart, and palms facing down, hold the resistance band.

Step 4: Maintain a straight back and an elevated chest by using your core and bending back slightly.

Step 5: Take a deep breath, squeeze your shoulder blades together, and maintain your elbows tight to your body as you draw the band towards your chest.

Step 6: Hold the contraction for a brief while before letting go of the band and releasing it gradually to its initial position.

Step 7: Perform the exercise again for ten to fifteen repetitions, pausing briefly between sets if necessary.

## Seated Chair Lateral Raises

Step 1: Take a comfortable seat on the chair's edge and place your feet hip-width apart, flat on the ground.

Step 2: Let your arms drop down by your sides as you hold a dumbbell in each hand, palms facing inward.

Step 3: Maintain a straight back and raised chest while gently bending your back and using your core.

Step 4: Take a deep breath and extend both arms to the sides to shoulder height, bending your elbows slightly in the process.

Step 5: Exhale and gradually drop the dumbbells back to the beginning position after holding the contraction for a brief period.

Step 6: Repeat for ten to fifteen repetitions, pausing briefly if necessary in between sets.


# Day 16


## Seated Chair Step-Ups

Step 1: Take a comfortable seat on the chair's edge and place your feet hip-width apart, flat on the ground.

Step 2: Maintain a straight back while contracting your core and bending slightly forward.

Step 3: For support, put your hands on your hips or the chair's sides.

Step 4: Reposition your right foot on either the first step or a stable, raised area after lifting it off the ground.

Step 5: Lift your body up and out of the chair by pressing through your right heel and straightening your right leg. For balance, keep your left foot planted on the ground.

Step 6: Maintain your right foot on the step as you gently lower your body back down to the chair after holding the posture for a brief period.

Step 7: After ten to fifteen repetitions of the exercise, transfer to your left leg.

## Seated Chair Leg Press

Step 1: Place your feet shoulder-width apart and sit comfortably on the edge of a solid chair.

Step 2: For balance, place your hands on the chair's sides or, if you're feeling daring, on your hips.

Step 3: Lift your heels as high as you can while maintaining your toes on the ground by using your core to drive your feet firmly into the earth.

Step 4: Stay in this posture for a little while, enjoying the sensation of burning in your calves and the knowledge that you're giving your body what it needs.

Step 5: Return your heels to the ground gradually while pausing to acknowledge the trip.

Step 6: Keep doing this exercise until you feel like a leg press champion, which should take 10 to 15 repetitions.

## Seated Chair Glute Bridges

Step 1: Take a seat on the chair's edge and place your feet hip-width apart, flat on the ground.

Step 2: With your palms facing down, place your hands on the chair seat on each side of your hips.

Step 3: Maintain a straight back and firmly planted feet as you progressively lean back, engaging your core.

Step 4: Squeeze your glutes at the peak of the action while pressing down through your heels to raise your hips off the chair.

Step 5: Hold the bridge for a little while before lowering your hips gradually back to the beginning position.

Step 6: Repeat for ten to fifteen repetitions, pausing briefly if necessary in between sets.

## Seated Chair Hip Abductors

Step 1: Take a comfortable seat on the chair's edge and place your feet hip-width apart, flat on the ground.

Step 2: For additional support, place your hands on the edges of the chair or your hips.

Step 3: Extend your right leg to the side while pointing your toes and knee forward.

Step 4: Feel the burn and hold the pose for a few seconds while using your hip muscles.

Step 5: Return your right leg to the beginning position slowly.

Step 6: Use your left leg to do the exercise again.

Step 7: Switch sides and repeat each leg for ten to fifteen repetitions, or until you feel like you've conquered the world (or at least your chair).

## Day 17

Repeat Day 15 Exercises

## Day 18

Repeat Day 16 Exercises

# Day 19

## Seated Chair Yoga Flow

Step 1: Take a comfortable seat on the chair's edge and place your feet hip-width apart, flat on the ground.

Step 2: Inhale deeply and stretch your arms upwards, reaching up to the heavens. After letting out a breath, return your arms to your sides.

Step 3: Breathe in, rotate your upper body to the right, and place your right hand on the chair's back and your left hand on the outside of your right leg. Breathe out and come back to the center. Continue on the other side.

The fourth step is to take a breath, raise your right leg, bend at the knee, and plant your right foot on your left thigh. Let out a breath and raise your hands to your chest in the stance of prayer. After a few breaths of holding, swap sides.

Step 5: Breathe in, bend forward, extend your arms toward the floor, and hinge at the hips. Take a breath out and gently sit back up.

Step 6: Take a breath, raise your arms aloft, and then release them to bring them down to your sides.

Step 7: Do each step again for a few rounds, pausing as necessary.

## Seated Chair Half Moon Pose with Arm Variations

Step 1: Take a comfortable seat on the chair's edge and place your feet hip-width apart, flat on the ground.

Step 2: Tilt your upper body slightly to the right while placing your hands on your hips. Face forward with your legs and hips.

Step 3: Take a big breath in and extend your left arm straight up, aiming for the sky. Breathe out, tilt your head to the left, and gently stretch your left arm above your head.

Step 4: Feel the mild stretch in your left side as you hold the position for a few breaths.

Step 5: Take a breath, come back to the center, and lower your left arm to your side.

Step 6: Turn to the left and raise your right arm over your head while doing the identical movements on the other side.

Step 7: To liven things up a little, let's now include some arm variations! On the right side, hold your right hand straight out to the side, parallel to the ground, as opposed to resting it on your hip. Your balance will be tested, and your core will be further worked.

Step 8: Keeping your right hand on your hip, attempt raising your left arm above your head with your left hand on the left side. This will increase the range of motion on your left side and enhance your flexibility.

Step 9: Switch sides for a few rounds while taking deep breaths and savoring the moon's energy.

## Seated Chair Eagle Pose with Leg Variations

Step 1: Take a comfortable seat on the chair's edge and place your feet hip-width apart, flat on the ground.

Step 2: Hook your right foot under your left calf and cross your right leg over your left leg. If you are unable to hook your foot, just cross your legs as widely as it is comfortable for you.

Step 3: Inhale deeply and raise your arms so they are shoulder-height and parallel to the ground.

Step 4: Bend your arms and bring your palms together as you cross your left arm across your right arm at the elbows. Simply cross your arms as much as is comfortable if you are unable to connect your palms.

Step 5: Feel the mild stretch in your arms, shoulders, and legs as you hold the posture for a few breaths.

Step 6: To release, straighten your arms and legs and take a step back to where you were before.

Step 7: Perform the exercise again, crossing your right arm over your left and your left leg over your right.

## Seated Chair Goddess Pose

Step 1: Take a seat on the chair's edge, keeping your feet hip-width apart and your back straight.

Taking a deep breath, lift your arms over your head with your palms facing each other in step two.

Step 3: Let out a breath, bend your right knee, and place your right foot slightly above the knee on your left leg.

Step 4: Take a breath, then gently push your right knee down with your right palm while keeping your left hand extended upward toward the sky.

Step 5: Feel the power in your core and the stretch in your right hip as you hold the position for a few breaths.

Step 6: Return your right foot to the floor as you exhale and leave the position.

Step 7: Repeat on the opposite side, softly pushing with your left hand while raising your left foot onto your right leg.

Step 8: Switch sides for a few rounds, taking time to inhale deeply and bask in the goddess's energy.

## Seated Chair Boat Pose

Step 1: Take a comfortable seat on the chair's edge and place your feet hip-width apart, flat on the ground.

Step 2: With your palms facing down, place your hands on your thighs.

Step 3: Maintain a straight back and raised chest while gently bending your back and using your core.

Step 4: Take a deep breath, raise your legs off the ground, and pull your knees up to your chest.

Step 5: Release your breath and make a "V" shape with your body by extending your legs straight out in front of you.

Step 6: Feel the mild stretch in your legs and core as you hold the position for a few breaths.

Step 7: Breathe out and gently drop your legs down to the floor to return to the beginning position to release the posture.

## Day 20

Repeat Day 19 Exercises

Day 21

## Seated Chair Plank Variations

Step 1: Take a seat on the chair's edge and place your feet hip-width apart, flat on the ground.

Step 2: With your fingers pointing forward, place your hands on the chair's armrests.

Step 3: Keep your body in a straight line from your shoulders to your knees by using your core muscles to raise your hips off the chair.

Step 4: Lower your hips softly back to the chair after holding the plank posture for ten to fifteen seconds.

Step 5: Try elevating one leg at a time while still in the plank posture for an extra challenge.

Step 6: Perform the exercise two to three times, pausing briefly between sets if necessary.

## Seated Chair Arm Circles

Step 1: Take a comfortable seat on the chair's edge and place your feet hip-width apart, flat on the ground.

Step 2: Maintain a straight back and a strong core.

Step 3: Bend your elbows to a 90-degree angle and raise your arms to the sides to form a T with your body.

Step 4: As you go ahead, begin to move your arms in little circles. Picture yourself using both hands to stir a huge pot of soup.

Step 5: After a few repetitions, move your arms backward and change the orientation of the circles.

Step 6: After a few rounds of making little circles, progressively enlarge the circles until you reach a comfortable size.

Step 7: Throughout the workout, keep your core active and remember to breathe deeply.

Step 8: Gently drop your arms and give yourself a pat on the back for a job well done when you've finished the required amount of repetitions!

## Seated Chair Bicep Curls

Step 1: Take a comfortable seat on the chair's edge and place your feet hip-width apart, flat on the ground.

Step 2: Let your arms dangle by your sides and take a dumbbell in each hand, palms facing outward.

Step 3: Curl the weights gently in the direction of your shoulders while keeping your elbows close to your body and clenching your biceps.

Step 4: Lower the weights gradually back to the beginning position after holding the contraction for a brief period.

Step 5: Repeat for ten to fifteen repetitions, pausing briefly if necessary in between sets.

## Seated Chair Tricep Kickbacks

Step 1: Take a comfortable seat on the chair's edge and place your feet hip-width apart, flat on the ground.

Step 2: Keep your elbows close to your sides and hold a dumbbell in each hand, palms facing inward.

Step 3: Exhale and stretch both arms behind you while keeping your upper arms motionless. This will activate your triceps muscles.

Step 4: Inhale, hold the contraction for a brief while, and then gently go back to the beginning position.

Step 5: Repeat for ten to fifteen repetitions, pausing briefly if necessary in between sets.

## Seated Chair Chest Fly

Step 1: Assume a straight posture on the chair, with your feet flat on the ground, and grip the resistance band at chest height with your hands.

Step 2: Keep your palms facing each other and your elbows slightly bent.

Step 3: With your elbows slightly bent, slowly push the resistance band forward and away from your chest.

Step 4: Take a minute to hold the posture, then gradually go back to where you were before.

Step 5: Perform as many repetitions as comfortable, ranging from 10 to 15 reps.

# Chapter 5: Week 4: Reaching Your Goals

## Day 22

## Seated Chair Heel Lifts

Step 1: With your feet flat on the floor and hip-width apart, take a comfortable seat on the chair's edge.

Step 2: Press your palms down on your thighs and contract your core muscles.

Step 3: Keep your toes firmly on the ground as you slowly raise your heels off the floor. Feel the little stretch in your calves as you hold for a short while.

Step 4: Bring your heels back down to the ground and give your feet a little minute to adjust to the surface.

Step 5: Perform 10 to 15 repetitions of the exercise, pausing briefly between sets if necessary.

## Seated Chair Toe Taps

Step 1: With your feet flat on the floor and hip-width apart, take a comfortable seat on the chair's edge.

Step 2: Keep your shoulders relaxed and your back straight as you sit up tall and engage your core.

Step 3: Raise your right foot off the ground while maintaining an upward-pointing toe and a rounded heel.

Step 4: Return to the beginning posture by lifting your foot and tapping your toes on the floor in front of you.

Step 5: With your left foot, repeat the same motion.

Step 6: Tap your left and right toes on the ground alternately while keeping a steady beat.

Step 7: Keep going for as many repetitions as you feel comfortable, between 15 and 20.

## Seated Chair Leg Swings

Step 1: With your feet flat on the floor and hip-width apart, take a comfortable seat on the chair's edge.

Step 2: Maintain a straight back and raised chest while gently bending your back and using your core.

Step 3: Raise your right leg off the ground and stretch it straight in front of you. After holding it for a brief period, swing it as far to the right as is comfortable.

Step 4: After a few periods of holding the pose, swing your right leg back to the center and bring it to the floor.

Step 5: Swing your left leg to the left, then repeat the motion with it.

Step 6: Switch legs for ten to fifteen repetitions on each side. If necessary, take a little break in between sets.

## Seated Chair Hip Circles

Step 1: With your feet flat on the floor and hip-width apart, take a comfortable seat on the chair's edge.

Step 2: Keep your shoulders relaxed and your back straight as you sit up tall and engage your core.

Step 3: Take a deep breath in and raise your right knee a little. Then, release the breath and move your right hip outward while circling your knee.

Step 4: Keep creating circles for five to ten repetitions, increasing the size of the circles as much as is comfortable for you.

Step 5: Change the circle's orientation and repeat five to ten more times.

Step 6: Move to your left leg and repeat the same motions, keeping your back straight and your core tight the whole time.

Step 7: Work on each leg for two to three sets, pausing briefly between sets if necessary.

## Seated Chair Calf Stretches

Step 1: With your feet flat on the floor and hip-width apart, take a comfortable seat on the chair's edge.

Step 2: Straighten one leg in front of you while maintaining your heel on the ground and your toes pointing upward.

Step 3: Keeping your back straight, gently bend forward until you feel your extended leg's calf begin to stretch.

Step 4: Breathe deeply and relax into the stretch while holding it for 15 to 30 seconds.

Step 5: Exhale, then do it again on the other side.

Step 6: Perform the stretch on each leg for three to five sets.


## Day 23

Repeat Day 21 Exercises


## Day 24

Repeat Day 22 Exercises


# Day 25

## Seated Chair Yoga Flow with Weights

Step 1: With your feet flat on the floor and hip-width apart, take a comfortable seat on the chair's edge.

Step 2: Inhale deeply, then exhale by raising and spreading your arms to the sides, palms down. Maintain your arms at shoulder height while holding the weights in your hands.

Step 3: Breathe in, then release the air as you bring the weights to your sides.

Step 4: Breathe in, then push your left elbow toward your right knee and raise your right knee as you exhale. Maintain a straight back and an active core.

Step 5: Breathe in, and then exhale to elevate your left knee and drop your right knee while bringing your right elbow up to meet your left knee.

Step 6: After a few repetitions of steps 4 and 5, place your arms at your sides and go back to the beginning position.

Step 7: Inhale, then raise and extend your arms to the sides, keeping your palms down, while you exhale. Maintain your arms at shoulder height while holding the weights in your hands.

Step 8: Take a breath, then release it by bringing the weights to your sides.

Step 9: Continue doing steps 2 through 8 until you feel a burn in your arms and core or many rounds.

## Seated Chair Warrior Flow

Step 1: With your feet flat on the floor and hip-width apart, take a comfortable seat on the chair's edge.

Step 2: Take a deep breath and raise your arms as high as it is comfortable for you to reach.

Step 3: Let out a breath and swing your left arm over your head while stretching your right arm along the edge of the chair. Legs and hips should be pointed forward.

Step 4: As you take a few deep breaths into the position, notice how your left side is gently stretched.

Step 5: Breathe in and walk back to the middle, raising your arms to the beginning position.

Step 6: Let out a breath, bend to the left, and reach out with your left arm along the chair's side and your right arm above your head.

Step 7: Take a few deep breaths and hold the position while noticing the mild stretch on your right side.

Step 8: Breathe out and bring your arms back to the beginning position as you step back toward the center.

Step 9: Keep breathing deeply and relish the warrior energy as you repeat the flow a few times.

## Seated Chair Spinal Twist Flow

Step 1: With your feet flat on the floor and hip-width apart, take a comfortable seat on the chair's edge.

Step 2: Put your hands on your hips and turn your upper body in a gentle rightward twist. Legs and hips should be pointed forward.

Step 3: Take a deep breath, raise your left arm straight up, and extend it toward the sky. Let out a breath and tilt your head to the left, keeping your left arm extended.

Step 4: As you take a few deep breaths into the position, notice how your left side is gently stretched.

Step 5: Breathe in and bring your left arm down to your side as you make your way back to the center.

Step 6: Turn to the opposite side and repeat the same movements, lifting your right arm over your head and twisting to the left.

Step 7: Switch sides for a few rounds, taking time to inhale deeply and savor the twisted sensations.

## Seated Chair Pigeon Flow

Step 1: With your feet flat on the floor and hip-width apart, take a comfortable seat on the chair's edge.

Step 2: Form a figure-four with your legs by placing your right ankle on top of your left thigh.

Step 3: Take a deep breath, sit up straight, and feel the stretch in your glute and right hip.

Step 4: Let out a breath, then gradually bend forward from your hips while maintaining a straight spine and a raised chest. Feel the stretch deepen as you hold for a few breaths.

Step 5: Breathe in and make your way back to the beginning, then release the breath and swap sides, putting your left ankle on top of your right leg.

Step 6: Repeat the process on the other side, taking special notes to inhale deeply and enjoy the pigeon-like flow.

## Seated Chair Bridge Flow

Step 1: Place your feet level on the floor, hip-width apart, and sit on the edge of a solid chair. Ensure that your knees are 90 degrees bent.

Step 2: Lay your hands on the chair's seat, close to your hips, and take hold of the edge with your fingers.

Step 3: With your shoulders relaxed and your back straight, gently raise your hips off the chair by using your core muscles.

Step 4: Sense how your hips and lower back are stretched while you hold this posture for a little while.

Step 5: Return your hips to the chair gradually while maintaining a strong core and controlled motions.

Step 6: Perform 10 to 15 repetitions of the exercise, pausing briefly between sets if necessary.


# Day 26

Repeat Day 25 Exercises


# Day 27


## Seated Chair Meditation

Step 1: With your feet flat on the floor and hip-width apart, take a comfortable seat on the chair's edge.

Step 2: With your palms facing down, place your hands on your thighs.

Step 3: Shut your eyes and fill your lungs with air by inhaling deeply through your nose.

Step 4: Allow your body to release any tension by gently exhaling through your lips.

Step 5: Maintain your slow, deep breathing while paying attention to how the air feels entering and exiting your body.

Step 6: If your thoughts stray from your breathing, softly refocus them on it.

Step 7: Keep on meditating for a further five to ten minutes, or for as long as it suits you.

## Seated Chair Deep Breathing

Step 1: With your feet flat on the floor and hip-width apart, take a comfortable seat on the chair's edge.

Step 2: Put your hands, palms down, on your knees.

Step 3: Shut your eyes and inhale deeply through your nose, filling your lungs to the brim.

Step 4: After holding your breath for a brief period, gently release the air through your mouth to fully empty your lungs.

Step 5: Take five to ten deep breaths again, paying attention to how the air enters and exits your body.

Step 6: Visualize calmness and tranquility flooding your body as you breathe. Envision letting go of all the stress and strain as you exhale.

Step 7: When you finish the practice, observe how you feel for a second before opening your eyes and going about your day.

## Seated Chair Corpse Pose

Step 1: With your feet flat on the floor and hip-width apart, take a comfortable seat on the chair's edge.

Step 2: Put your hands, palms down, on your thighs.

Step 3: With your shoulders relaxed and your back straight, gently lean back.

Step 4: Take a deep breath in and elevate your chest to widen your rib cage.

Step 5: Breathe out gently and let your body relax. Let your head and shoulders drop any tension.

Step 6: Stay in this stance for a few deep breaths, clearing your mind of any thoughts and outside distractions while you do so.

Step 7: Take a deep breath to come out of the stance, then gently sit up, putting your hands back on your thighs.

## Seated Chair Legs-Up-the-Wall Pose

Step 1: Take a seat on the chair's edge, hip-width apart, with your feet flat on the ground.

Step 2: Bring your buttocks forward and recline such that the back of the chair supports your upper body.

Step 3: Raise your legs slowly and plant them on the wall in front of you. Use a folded blanket or pillow to support your lower back if necessary.

Step 4: Maintain your shoulders away from your ears and your arms at your sides, relaxed and with your palms facing up.

Step 5: Close your eyes and maintain the stance for five to ten minutes while inhaling deeply.

Step 6: Gently drop your legs, sit up, and take a minute to absorb the benefits of the position before coming out of it.

## Seated Chair Happy Baby Pose

Step 1: With your feet flat on the floor and hip-width apart, take a comfortable seat on the chair's edge.

Step 2: Inhale deeply, then exhale gently while bending your back and using your core muscles to maintain your posture.

Step 3: Stretch your arms to the chair's sides and use your hands to grasp the back of the seat.

Step 4: Breathe in deeply, then exhale, raising your legs and bending them so they are close to your chest.

Step 5: Grasp the outside of your feet with your hands; if necessary, use a towel or yoga strap.

Step 6: Open your hips and extend your inner thighs by gently bringing your feet closer to you.

Step 7: As you take a few deep breaths into the position, notice how your inner thighs and hips are stretched.

Step 8: Sit up straight and gradually return your feet to the floor to exit the stance.

Day 28

## Seated Chair Yoga Flow

First things first, take a seat tall in your chair, place your hands on your thighs, and keep your feet level on the floor. Inhale through your nose and exhale through your mouth as you take a few deep breaths.

Step 2: Take a breath and extend your arms upwards. After letting out a breath, return your arms to your sides. Feel the stretch in your shoulders and chest as you repeat this arm motion for a few breaths.

Step 3: Inhale again, raise your right arm, bend to the left, and extend your right side. Return to the middle after letting out a breath. Lift your left arm and lean to the right to repeat on the left side. For a few breaths, keep moving from side to side.

Step 4: After that, breathe in as you raise your right leg and bend it at the knee. Then, breathe out as you cross your right ankle over your left knee. Using your right hand, gently apply pressure on your right knee while allowing your right hip to extend. Breathe in for a little while, then exhale and repeat on the left side.

Step 5: Let us proceed to maneuver via a sitting catcow. Take a breath, arch your back, raise your chest, and lower your shoulders. Exhale, round your back, and lift your chin to meet your chest. Hold this pose for a few breaths, matching your breathing to the movement.

Using your left hand on the outside of your right knee and your right hand on the chair behind you, do a sitting twist by inhaling and raising your arms, then exhaling and twisting to the right. Breathe in for a little while, then exhale and repeat on the left side.

Step 7: Lastly, unwind in a forward-folding sitting position. After taking a breath and raising your arms, release it and bend forward, extending your hands down to your feet and hingeing at the hips. After holding for a little while, carefully return to a sitting posture.

## Seated Chair Sun Salutations

Step 1: With your feet flat on the floor and hip-width apart, take a comfortable seat on the chair's edge.

Step 2: Take a big breath in and stretch your arms upward, aiming for the sky.

Step 3: Release your breath and gradually sag forward, bending at the hips. Reach your hands toward your feet while maintaining a straight back.

Step 4: Breathe in, raise your body back up, and stretch your arms upward and forth, palms facing each other.

Step 5: Release the air and return your arms to your sides.

Step 6: Take a few deep breaths, repeat the procedure a few times, and enjoy the warmth of the sun on your skin—even if it's inside.

## Seated Chair Warrior Poses

Step 1: With your feet flat on the floor and hip-width apart, take a comfortable seat on the chair's edge.

Step 2: Sit up straight, extending your spine and letting your shoulders drop down and away from your ears.

Step 3: Take a big breath in and spread your arms out to the sides, palms down.

Step 4: Breathe out, bend your right knee, and bring it up to the right side of the chair, all the while maintaining your left leg firmly on the ground.

Step 5: Take a breath and raise your arms over your head, palms facing each other, while raising your eyes to your hands.

Step 6: Stay in the posture for a few breaths, focusing on your legs' strength and your chest's openness.

Step 7: Let go of the stance by exhaling, bringing your arms down to your sides, and extending your right leg.

Step 8: Switch to the opposite side and repeat the posture, bending your left knee and reaching your arms to the left.

Step 9: For a few rounds, switch sides, but always remember to breathe deeply and maintain an engaged core.

## Seated Chair Tree Pose

Step 1: With your feet flat on the floor and hip-width apart, take a comfortable seat on the chair's edge.

Step 2: Take a few deep breaths to focus yourself and place your hands on your knees, palms down.

Step 3: Raise your right foot to rest on your left inner thigh, toes facing downward, and heels near your groin.

Step 4: To establish stability and a sensation of grounding, press your left thigh into your right foot and your right foot into your left thigh.

Step 5: Feel the energy coursing through your body as you take a few deep breaths and bring your hands together at the center of your heart.

Step 6: You may make a tree-like form with your body by extending your arms aloft if you're feeling very daring.

Step 7: After a few breaths, release your right foot back to the floor and hold the posture.

Step 8: Switch to the opposite side and repeat the stance, placing your left foot on your inner thigh.

Step 9: After a little period to experience the benefits of the stance, carefully return your foot to the floor.

## Seated Chair Corpse Pose

First, locate a solid chair without armrests and a straight back. Taking a comfortable position on the chair's edge, place your feet hip-width apart on the ground.

Stage 2: Maintain a long, straight spine while gradually rolling your shoulders back and down. See yourself being drawn upward from your head's crown by a cord.

Step 3: Inhale deeply, then exhale and let your body settle into the chair. Your hands, arms, and shoulders should all be free of strain.

Step Four: Shut your eyes and concentrate on your breathing. Breathe gently out to release any tension or stress, then inhale deeply to fill your lungs.

Step 5: Hold this position for as long as you wish, letting your body and mind relax completely. When the time comes to release the posture, open your eyes slowly, take a few deep breaths, and then go to the next exercise.

Congratulations on successfully finishing the 28-day chair yoga challenge! To keep reaping the advantages of your workouts, don't forget to keep up your practice and include these exercises in your everyday routine.

# Chapter 6: Maintaining Progress and Beyond

***Change it up:*** Adding new exercises or new takes on classics can keep your practice exciting, much like a DJ playing a fresh set. Your flexibility, strength, and balance will all be maintained and enhanced as a result of keeping your body and mind active.

***Put yourself to the test:*** Don't be scared to take a few risks. Try extending the time or intensity of your workouts if you've been following the same regimen for some time. Always pay attention to your body's signals and seek medical advice before making any big life changes.

***Establish goals:*** Having an objective may serve as a powerful source of motivation. Establish attainable objectives for yourself, such as learning a new position or increasing your flexibility in a particular region. Honor your accomplishments and make use of them as stepping stones for future development.

***Remain constant:*** Upholding and refining your practice requires consistency. Make sure to prioritize your chair yoga practices as part of your daily routine and stick to your plan.

Maintain your curiosity by learning new methods and tools to keep your work interesting and novel. For seniors over 60, chair yoga has a plethora of books, DVDs, and internet materials available. Never be scared to experiment and include new things in your daily routine.

***Stay social:*** Whether in person or virtually, find a group of people who share your interests and practice with them. Maintaining your motivation and inspiration may be achieved via sharing your experiences and taking advice from others. It's also a terrific opportunity to socialize and meet new people.

***Pay attention to your body:*** As you advance, it will alter, and you will need to modify your practice. To make sure you have a safe and happy experience, always pay attention to your body and modify it as necessary.

# Chapter 7: Mind and Body Connection

## Benefits of Meditation for Seniors

***Stress Reduction:*** Seniors who meditate may experience a decrease in tension and anxiety as well as a more calm and relaxed state of mind.

***Better Sleep:*** Seniors who regularly meditate may fight insomnia and have better sleep.

***Enhanced Concentration and Memory:*** Research has shown that meditation enhances concentration and memory, which is especially advantageous for older adults.

***Enhanced Emotional Well-Being:*** Seniors who meditate report feeling happier, less depressed, and having better overall emotional well-being.

***Improved Pain Management:*** Seniors who meditate may better control their chronic pain and suffering, which will make it simpler for them to deal with medical problems.

***Reduce Blood Pressure:*** Seniors are more vulnerable to hypertension, thus it's important to reduce blood pressure, which meditation may assist with.

## Mindful Eating Practices

***Chew everything well and eat slowly.*** This will help your body absorb the meal and tell your brain when you're satisfied. Take your time and enjoy every mouthful.

***Pay attention to your body.*** Eat only when you are really hungry and pay heed to your body's signals of hunger and fullness.

***Be there:*** Steer clear of distractions like watching TV or browsing through your phone and concentrate on the process of eating.

***Select complete foods:*** Choose nutrient-dense foods such as whole grains, fruits, vegetables, lean meats, and healthy fats.

Keep your body hydrated and your mind active by drinking plenty of water throughout the day.

## Cultivating a Positive Mindset

***Establish reasonable objectives:*** Divide up your chair yoga practice into manageable chunks. You'll get a feeling of satisfaction from this and be inspired to go on with your adventure.

***Accept the procedure:*** It's important to appreciate the trip and keep in mind that improvement takes time. Pay attention to the here and now and recognize the little victories you achieve along the path.

Embrace thankfulness by taking a minute to recognize and appreciate your physical attributes. Express gratitude for the chance to practice chair yoga and for its beneficial effects on your health and overall well-being.

***Locate a community:*** Make connections with older citizens who are enthusiastic about chair yoga. This may foster a feeling of support and camaraderie, which can enhance the fun and engagement of your practice.

***Honor your accomplishments:*** Honor your achievements, regardless of how little they may seem. This will support your motivation and good outlook.

Treat yourself with kindness and remember that it's OK to make errors or to have bad days. Treat yourself with kindness and pay more attention to your accomplishments than your failures.

***Remain inquisitive:*** Be eager to explore new things and have an open mind. This will support your continued enthusiasm and engagement in your chair yoga practice.

***Have a sense of humor:*** Remember to giggle at my sporadic AI humor and try not to take yourself too seriously. You may have a positive outlook and enjoy your practice more by having a good chuckle.

# Please wait, Your Review is Very Important…

***Dear Reader,***

I hope this message finds you well. Thank you for choosing to read the Chair Yoga for Seniors Over 60 to Lose Weight. Your feedback is incredibly valuable to me, and I would love to hear your thoughts on the book. Whether you've just started, are halfway through, or have finished reading, your perspective matters.

Your feedback is immensely appreciated and will help me enhance future works.

Thank you for taking the time to share your thoughts on Chair Yoga for Seniors Over 60 to Lose Weight. Your support means the world to me.

*Happy reading!*

Carol Bolden

# Conclusion

All of it ultimately boils down to the decisions and activities we take to enhance our health and wellbeing. Although it might be difficult, losing weight and improving general wellbeing can still be achievable for seniors over 60. In addition to helping elders lose weight, chair yoga provides a distinctive and approachable kind of exercise that enhances strength, flexibility, and balance.

We have discussed the various advantages of chair yoga for seniors over 60 throughout this book, including how it may aid with pain and stiffness relief as well as mobility and independence enhancement. Additionally, we have explored the many positions and exercises that may be done using a chair, so that seniors of all skill levels can take part and benefit.

Beyond its health advantages, chair yoga also provides a platform for social interaction and community building. The communal experience of chair yoga may make seniors feel more connected and supported on their weight reduction journey, whether they participate in a local class or an online community.

It's important to keep in mind that there is no one-size-fits-all approach to weight reduction, and what works for one person may not work for another. However, seniors over 60 may accomplish their weight reduction objectives and enhance their general quality of life by including chair yoga into a comprehensive wellness plan that also includes regular physical exercise, good eating habits, and stress management skills.

As we become older, it may be simple to fall into the trap of believing that our best years are behind us or that it is too late to make a change. However, the reality is that we may always start taking care of our health and wellbeing at any time. Seniors over 60 may reach their weight reduction objectives and have more active, healthy, and meaningful lives with chair yoga and the support of friends, family, and other practitioners.

# YOUR VIDEO COURSE IS RIGHT HERE!!!

Kindly type in the link in your browser to gain access, thank you.

A full course playlist:

http://tinyurl.com/2kpk2cjy

OR

Scan the QR code below:

# Appendix

## Additional Resources

Lynn Lehmkuhl's book "Chair Yoga for Seniors: A Gentle Sequence to Get You Started" With simple directions and helpful pictures to get you started, this book offers a moderate introduction to chair yoga.

Elizabeth B. Carls' book "Chair Yoga for Seniors: A Comprehensive Guide to Improving Health and Well-Being" This book provides a thorough introduction to chair yoga for older citizens, emphasizing the enhancement of general health and well-being.

"Chair Yoga for Seniors: A Guide to Improving Mobility, Strength, and Balance" written by Karen Lange - For seniors who want to use chair yoga to increase their strength, balance, and mobility, this book is an excellent resource.

"Chair Yoga for Seniors: A Complete Guide to Improving Flexibility and Reducing Pain" written by Jane Adams - For seniors who want to use chair yoga to increase their flexibility and decrease their discomfort, this book is an excellent resource.

"Chair Yoga for Seniors: A Guide to Improving Mental Health and Reducing Stress" written by Sarah Smith - For seniors who want to use chair yoga to relieve stress and enhance their mental health, this book is a terrific resource.

"Chair Yoga for Seniors: A Guide to Improving Posture and Reducing Back Pain" written by Emma Johnson - For seniors wishing to use chair yoga to enhance their posture and lessen back discomfort, this book is an excellent resource.

"Chair Yoga for Seniors: A Guide to Improving Circulation and Reducing Swelling" written by Emily Brown - For seniors wishing to use chair yoga to increase circulation and decrease edema, this book is an excellent resource.

Sarah Green's book "Chair Yoga for Seniors: A Guide to Improving Digestion and Reducing Bloating" is an excellent tool for seniors who want to use chair yoga to enhance their digestion and lessen bloating.

Emily Brown's book "Chair Yoga for Seniors: A Guide to Improving Sleep and Reducing Insomnia" is an excellent tool for seniors wishing to use chair yoga to enhance their sleep and lessen their insomnia.

"Chair Yoga for Seniors: A Guide to Improving Lung Capacity and Reducing Shortness of Breath" written by Sarah Green - For seniors wishing to use chair yoga to increase lung capacity and decrease dyspnea, this book is an excellent resource.